D1036446

Sanctuary

Renewing the Rhythm of Rest & Renewal

Gloria J. Burgess

SECOND EDITION

Sanctuary

Renewing the Rhythm of Rest & Renewal

Also by Gloria J. Burgess

Books

Pass It On!

*Flawless Leadership: Connecting Who You Are
with What You Know and Do*

The Embodiment of Leadership (editor)

Leading in Complex Worlds (editor)

Dare to Wear Your Soul on the Outside: Live Your Legacy Now

*Legacy Living: The Six Covenants for Personal &
Professional Excellence*

Continuum: The First Songbook of Sweet Honey in the Rock (editor)

Poetry

Journey of the Rose

The Open Door

A Yellow Wood

Sanctuary

Renewing the Rhythm of Rest & Renewal

Gloria J. Burgess

Red Oak Press
Edmonds, Washington

Sanctuary
Restoring the Rhythm of Rest & Renewal
Gloria J. Burgess

Red Oak Press
Edmonds, Washington

Cover Design: Terren Sky Krietzman
Photography Editor: Lucas Oncina
Editorial/Production: Jan B. Seymour
Author Photo: Richard Brummett
Pages 30-33 Background Art: Terren Sky Krietzman
All quotes without attribution: Gloria J. Burgess

ISBN: 978-1-892864-06-2
Printed in the USA

To John

My soulmate and best friend who supports me
in making a way for sanctuary
and—most importantly—practicing what I preach!

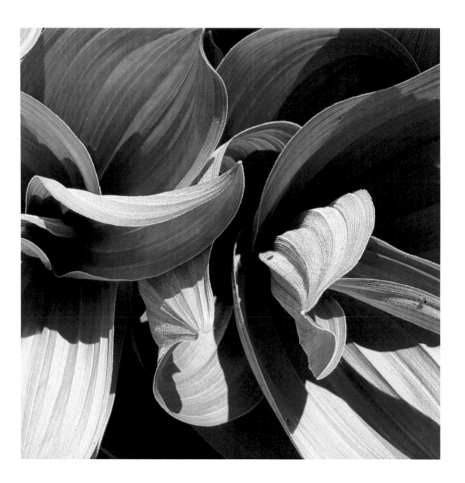

Table of Contents

Inside myself is a place where I live all alone and that is where I renew my springs that never dry up.

PEARL S. BUCK

Rest is the original transformative technology. Through rest we rebuild, rewire, and renew ourselves—literally.

MATTHEW EDLUND, M.D.

Thank you is the best prayer that anyone could say. I say that one a lot. Thank you expresses extreme gratitude, humility, understanding.

ALICE WALKER

Though a tree grow ever so high, the falling leaves return to the ground.

MALAY PROVERB

How we spend our days is, of course, how we spend our lives.

ANNIE DILLARD

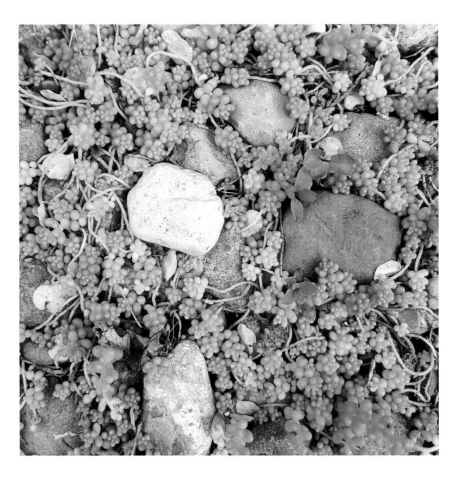

Introduction

We have all experienced sanctuary at some time in
our lives.

Many of you will recognize sanctuary as an intentional
time out, a purposeful pause from your normal stream of
continuous activity. You will move through these pages
with ease and with a sense, however faint, of the familiar.

That sense is your innate knowing of the sacred.
It is your soul's remembrance of who you are.
Who you are when you're not over-committed.
Who you are when you're not overwhelmed.
Who you are when you're not obsessed with speed.
Who you are when you're not distracted.
Who you are when you're not stressed out.
Who you are when you're not numbed out.
Who you are when you're not merely going
through the motions of living.

Instead… you are living the life that is meant *just for you*.
A life that embraces and seamlessly includes the natural,
necessary rhythms of rest and renewal.

A few of you might flee from the very mention
of sanctuary.

Resist that urge.

Instead, consider this book as a gentle summons,
a gracious reminder that is calling to you.

Calling to you to let go.

> Calling to you to simply pause… and
> surrender to a slower tempo, to a pace and
> rhythm that is altogether different from your
> frenetic daily routine.

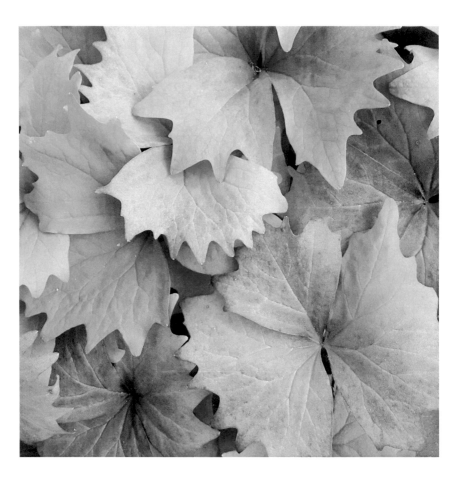

Gratitudes

I'm grateful for my amazing collaborators: Jan Seymour for her editorial and prepress excellence and two of my youthful mentors—Terren for his refreshing design and Lucas for his beautiful photography.

I'm grateful for the people in my life who have held, mentored, and nurtured me—family, friends, and total strangers who have helped me learn more deeply about sanctuary, its profound necessity and beneficial balm in our speed-obsessed culture.

I'm grateful for the healing presences of place and the powerful guidance and sustenance of the Holy Spirit.

I'm also grateful to you for caring enough about yourself and those you love to learn about sanctuary.

And finally, my deep gratitude to all the people and places that continue to reveal the blessings of sanctuary.

Archbishop Emeritus
Desmond Tutu • Billye Avery •
Cape Coast, Ghana • Cape Town, South Africa
Chamonix, France • Chartres Cathedral • Cortes Island,
British Columbia • Dalai Lama • Derek Walcott • Eva & Ron
Sher • Flam, Norway • Frederic Brussat • Glacier National Park
Grand Canyon • Henri Nouwen • Hildegarde de Bingen • J. Rosamond
Johnson • Jalāl al-Dīn Muhammad Rūmī • James Weldon Johnson •
Jerusalem, Israel • Jesus • Jill Geoffrion • Joan Chittester • John Lane
John O'Donohue • Joshua Tree National Monument • Joy Harjo • Kahlil
Gibran • Kakamanga Forest (Kenya) • Kathleen Norris • Kauai, Hawaii
King David • Lauren Artress • Le Mont Saint-Michel • Lois Greenberg
M. J. Ryan • Madeleine L'Engle • Mary Ann Brussat • Mary Oliver •
Meister Eckhardt • Mildred Blackmon McEwen • Molokai, Hawaii •
Mother Teresa • Mount Rainier • Naomi Shihab Nye • Neah Bay,
Washington • Niagara Falls • Notre Dame Cathedral • Pam Grout •
Patrice Vecchione • Quinault Rainforest • Redwood National Forest
Sagrada Familia • Saint Francis of Assisi • Saint Paul • Sainte-
Chapelle • Salisbury Cathedral • Salisbury Plain • Salish Sea
Sleeping Bear Dunes • Susan L. Taylor • Thomas Merton
Thomas Moore • Tuscany (Italy) • Waldron Island,
Washington • Wales • Washington National
Cathedral • Wendy Beckett • Whidbey
Island, Washington

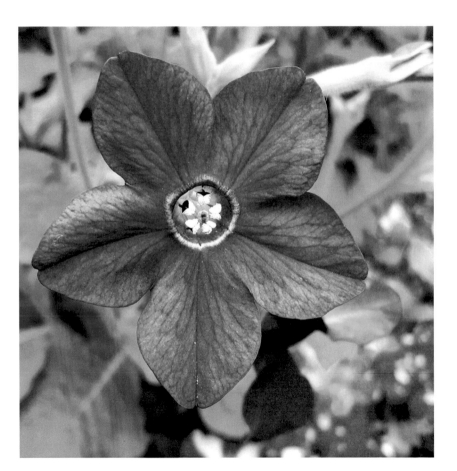

Sanctuary: *Experience the Eternal*

In Kairos *we are, we are fully in isness… fully, wholly, positively.*
MADELEINE L'ENGLE

Sanctuary resides within. It dwells in our innermost being. The many blessings that sanctuary offers include respite, rest, renewal, re-ignition, and restoration.

That *sanctuary resides within* runs counter to the common belief that sanctuary is some*thing* that exists outside of ourselves.

Sanctuary is not a thing. However, certain experiences and physical places can provide clues about the feeling tone of the sanctuary within: a long walk, breathtaking sunsets, mountains, cathedrals, forests, deserts, meadows, labyrinths, lakes, beautiful refuges of our own making. Having experienced such environs, we instinctively know they can evoke the feeling tone of sanctuary. And they can also enhance our awareness of how we can cultivate sanctuary as an interior resource.

The key challenge to experiencing sanctuary is to make the transition from doing to being. To make this shift, you must let go of your busyness in the exterior realm of doing *so that* you can cross the threshold and enter your interior realm of being.

This means letting go of your ordinary life to enter the extraordinary realm of sanctuary. A realm of rest and renewal, wonder and revelation where your emotional, intellectual, physical, and spiritual health and happiness are primary.

In other words, you must let go of serving others—just for a while, just for *you*—so you can be of service to yourself.

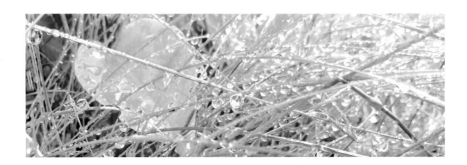

When you attend to and care for your interior life,
you will reap rewards in your exterior life.

For some of you, your inner sanctuary is readily accessible. Like a dear friend, it is an abiding, familiar, and palpable presence.

And when you're out of harmony, you simply access your inner sanctuary to help you remember who you are. You attune to the sacred whispers within to recenter yourself, to welcome yourself home to your own true nature.

For others, sanctuary is obscured, hidden.

Perhaps it's buried beneath the mound of life-draining drama, disappointments, and distractions you have allowed to invade and inhabit your interior life. And now, you must divine, uncover, and reacquaint yourself with your inner sanctuary.

Whether it is your constant companion or hidden deep within you, sanctuary beckons you to liberate yourself from distraction, exhaustion, and overwork… to step away from the oppressive demands of clock time.

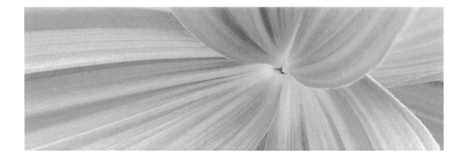

Sanctuary summons you to cross the threshold into the gracious realm of tranquility and refreshment where the daily tyranny of hours and minutes and seconds no longer rule.

This summons is an exquisite invitation.
An invitation to step out
of the ordinary and enter
into *Kairos*—that extraordinary experience
of the eternal—that lives
and breathes within you.

Sanctuary invites you to immerse yourself in this extraordinary time out of time, an ample presence you can cultivate and take with you wherever you go.

Notes

Notes

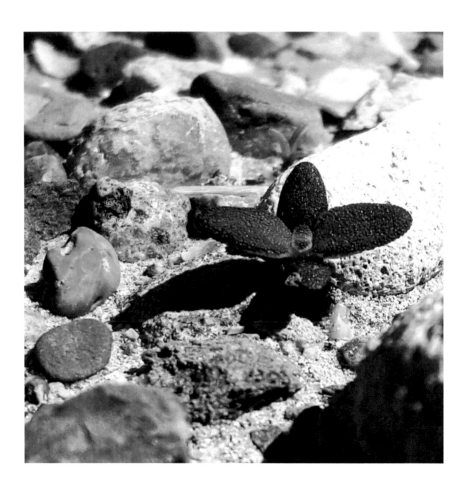

2

Seeking Sanctuary

Sanctuary is your soul's reason for being.
ANONYMOUS

Seeking sanctuary requires us to slow down. In our culture of speed, slowing down is not the norm. Slowing down is actually countercultural.

So, seeking and saying *yes* to sanctuary is a radical act. It is a radical act of hospitality. Indeed, it is one of the marvelous ways we can inwardly proclaim and host the majesty of our soul.

Like any other form of artistry,
proclaiming your soul is
a political act, a revolutionary
offering of bread and water
to the hungry and thirsty in spirit.

A way to begin to seek sanctuary is to notice those places and spaces and people and moments that nourish you. That refresh you. That revive you. A warm breeze brushing your face. Falling asleep beneath a star-studded sky. Gazing out upon a tranquil sea. Relaxing in your favorite chair in a secluded spot in your own backyard. Listening to soothing or uplifting music. Enjoying the sacred pause of life-affirming silence. Unplugging from your iPad or cell phone for an entire day. A long, quiet stroll in the park.

You can also seek sanctuary by noticing what awakens your senses. By noticing what reinvigorates and renews you. Colors. Fragrances. Images. Shapes. Sounds. Tastes. Textures. Silence.

As you heighten your awareness of your sensory environment, you are actually equipping yourself to notice, nourish, and nurture the sanctuary that resides within you. As you seek sanctuary, you are actually cultivating some of the habits, or practices, of sanctuary. In Chapter 4, I include a number of other practices to cultivate sanctuary.

For now, notice the rhythm of your daily and weekly routines. Ask yourself: *What nourishes me? What renews and rejuvenates me? What helps me feel rested and restored? What helps me feel fully alive and present?*

Jot down your responses. Your answers to these questions provide clues to experiencing, seeking, and cultivating sanctuary.

They provide clues to what feeds and nourishes your soul.

When you acknowledge
and claim your soul,
you assert authority and power
in your life.

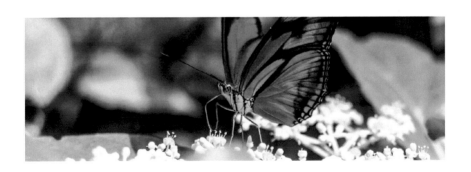

We all long for a way of being that has affinity with the soul. An affinity that opens us to experience the present moment with immediacy, intention, and emotion.

Appreciating the sun's warm caress on a beautiful summer morning.

Enjoying the relaxation and rhythm of play.

Loving yourself for who you are.

Engaging in radiant relationships with family and friends.

Sanctuary nurtures our affinity with soul, allowing you to:

Splurge in your senses.

See with new eyes.

Listen deeply.

Appreciate the miracle of each new day.

Open new doors.

See beyond differences.

Embrace our shared humanity.

Be a global citizen.

Engage in purposes beyond your own.

Believe in someone else's future.

Belong to lives other than your own.

Respect the birthright dignity of all.

Be guided by a power older than civilization or culture, older than time.

Lift your eyes to a horizon beyond your day-to-day routine.

Enjoy the realm of sanctuary!

Rest, renew, and restore yourself.

Re-ignite your passion.

Reconnect with your purpose.

Remember all that is essential.

Recatalyze your life force energy.

Rejoice in your innate gifts of awe, creativity, imagination, inspiration, joy, and wonder.

Re-enchant your life.

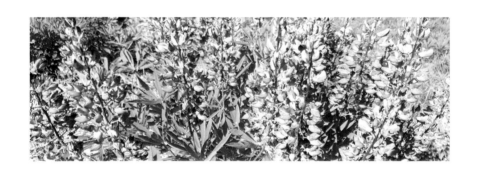

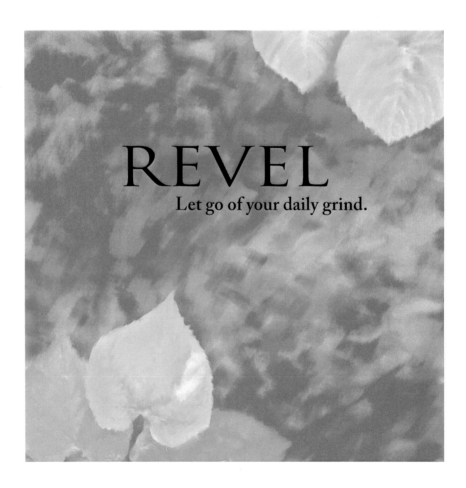

REVEL

Let go of your daily grind.

REJOICE
Remember who you are.

RENEW
Reflect on your own true nature.

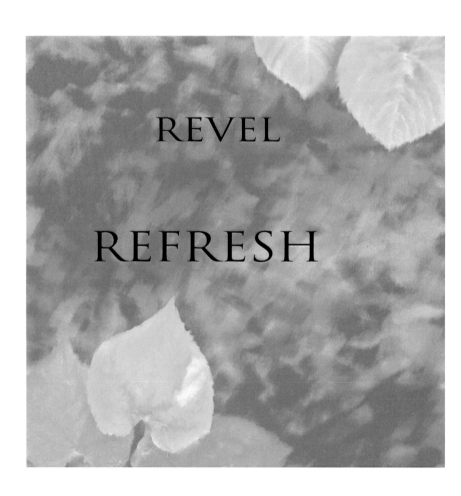

REVEL

REFRESH

REJOICE

RENEW

REJUVENATE

Notes

Notes

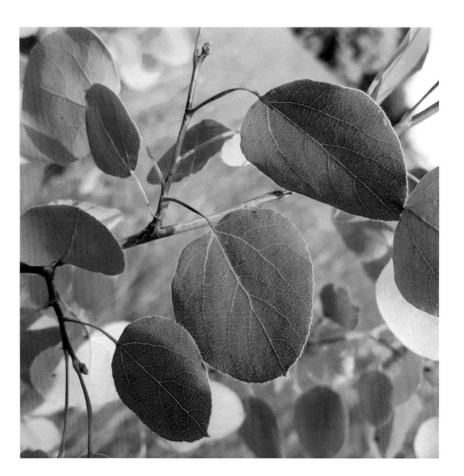

3

Making Way for *Sanctuary*

Humans are profoundly rhythmic. It's the main way we communicate, through both language and music.
MATTHEW EDLUND, M.D.

Sanctuary calls us to get centered and grounded, so we can attune to and tend to the parts of ourselves that are frazzled, out of sync, or just plain fried.

In our hectic, fast-paced lives, we all need to pause for refreshment and renewal.

Without pauses, or rests, what we call music would be nothing more than a continuous stream of white noise.

The same is true in our lives.

Without pausing, without rest, the grand symphony of our life becomes nothing more than a continuous stream of meaningless activity.

When we pause, we make way for sanctuary. This sacred pause provides gracious space for us to pay attention to the magnificent music of our lives. This sacred pause provides food to nourish our souls.

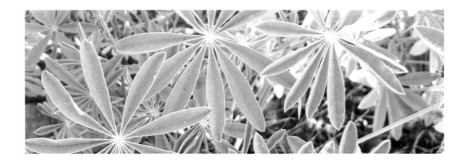

Notice the song in your own heart. That song is your unique melody. Your melody is all about your why. Your unique reason for being alive.

Sanctuary invites you to ask yourself: *Am I singing my own song? Or, am I singing someone else's song?* In other words, *am I being true to my unique purpose?*

Notice how you connect with others. That's your harmony, which is all about how you relate, connect, and engage with family, friends, co-workers, neighbors, animals, plants, and our planet.

Sanctuary invites you to ask yourself: *Am I living only for myself? Am I in tune with my spouse? My kids? Am I connecting with my classmates or team members or friends? Am I a good neighbor? When I reach out to others, how might I serve them while also being faithful to myself?*

Notice your pace, your tempo. Is it fast or slow or is it just right?

Sanctuary invites you to ask yourself: *Am I going so fast that I lose track of who and what is important to me?* In other words, *do I stop and smell the roses? Do I include time for friends and other loved ones? Or, am I going so slow that I miss out on moments, opportunities, and relationships?*

Notice your cadence, or rhythm. Your rhythm is all about who and what you value. It's about who and what you put in the center of your life. Or on the sidelines.

Sanctuary invites you to ask yourself: *Who do I include? Who do I exclude? Do I pay attention to who and what has heart and meaning? What do I emphasize? How does this serve me and others? What new rhythms must I learn for this season of my life?*

When we are in concert with the music of our lives—our melody, harmony, tempo, and rhythm—we attend to the condition and resonance of our own soul. And, at the same time, we attend to the condition and resonance of the world soul, this wondrous Global Village we call home.

When we are attuned to the music of our lives, we can reconnect to our highest calling.

In the exterior realm of doing, it is all too easy to get off track and lose your groove, to get out of alignment and be out of harmony with yourself and with your calling.

In this realm of doing, there is much that conspires against you:

Competing priorities.

Distractions.

Limiting beliefs.

Self-sufficiency.

Multi-tasking.

Old patterns.

Other people's agendas for you.

Your own insecurities, critical judgments, and so much more. What else would you add?

_____

_____

_____

_____

_____

_____

_____

threshold | noun | thresh•old | \'thresh-hōld

An opening that allows you
to walk away from the territory
of external demands and step into
a realm of inner freedom.

Sanctuary beckons you to cross the threshold from doing to being. When you cross that threshold, five important resources await you: *intention, commitment, compassion, humility,* and *joy.* When you draw on these spiritual resources, their blessings are immeasurable.

Each resource is an invitation to make way for sanctuary.

INTENTION

The first invitation is to consciously set your intention. Intention offers the twin gifts of clarity and focus.

When you set your intention to make a way for sanctuary, this life-affirming action will ensure a difference today and a different tomorrow.

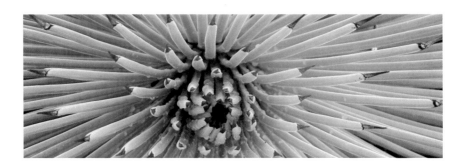

Light a candle to remind yourself that setting your intention is a sacred moment. Lighting a candle is a time-honored way to bring light into darkness. To bring light into a broken world. In this way, you focus your attention on what truly matters.

Intention is the antidote
to distraction.

COMMITMENT

Commitment is about dedication and faithfulness.

The invitation is to commit to your own wellbeing.

Making an intentional commitment to your own wellbeing is a special gift. A gift from you and for you.

This gift draws you into an oasis of self-love and self-care. Here, you can refresh yourself in the sacred waters of awe, beauty, humor, joy, play, silence, solitude, and wonder.

On a notepad, small sheet of paper, or sticky note, write: *I commit to my own wellbeing*. Put your note in a place where you will see it throughout the day. Do this for the next 30 days.

Commitment turns vision into volition.

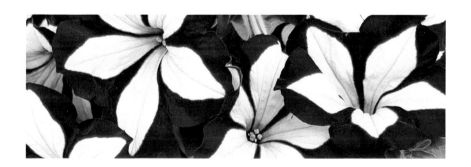

COMPASSION

Compassion is about being aware and caring and kind. It's also about being courageous, about being willing to help others who are suffering.

Compassion invites you to begin with yourself, which is a wondrous gift. Beginning with yourself opens your heart to have compassion and mercy for others.

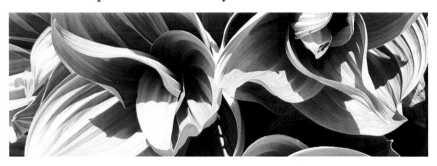

Find a few things around your home or office that are heart shaped. I enjoy collecting heart-shaped rocks. Over the years, I've received gifts of hearts shaped from wood, onyx, and soapstone. I also love photos of plants with heart-shaped leaves: anthurium, beech, hosta, morning glory, violets.

Take a picture of your favorite heart shape. Keep it as a reminder as your own heart opens to have greater compassion for yourself and others.

Love and compassion are necessities, not luxuries.
Without them humanity cannot survive.
Dalai Lama

HUMILITY

Humility is not thinking any more or less of yourself than you think of anyone else. In other words, you value and honor yourself the same as others.

Humility invites you to ask yourself: *How can I support my own health and happiness in this moment?*

One of the many gifts of humility is inspiration. Inspire comes from *inspirare*, which means to breathe into or upon. When we are inspired, we are infused with life from a force outside of ourselves.

On your daily or weekly to-do list, be sure to include your own name. Write *sanctuary* next to your name. Now, be sure your name and *sanctuary* are at the top of your list.

What humility does for one is
it reminds us that there are people before me.

MAYA ANGELOU

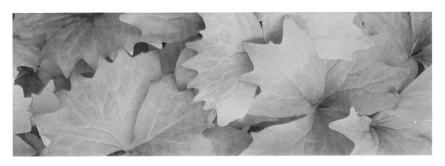

JOY

The invitation of joy is to recognize the divinity within you.

Sometimes we confuse happiness and joy.

 Happiness comes from outside.

 Joy comes from within.

 Happiness is a free-flowing stream.

 Joy is white-water exhilaration.

 Happiness is often fleeting.

 Joy is constant.

True joy, a precious gift, comes from the satisfaction of being content with and faithful to who and whose you are.

Celebrate yourself. Sing your favorite song. Dance like no one is watching.

Joy is the infallible sign of the presence of God.

Pierre Teilhard de Chardin

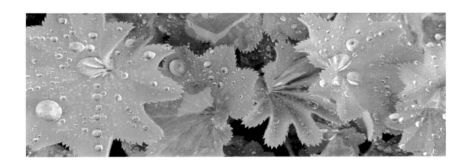

Notes

Notes

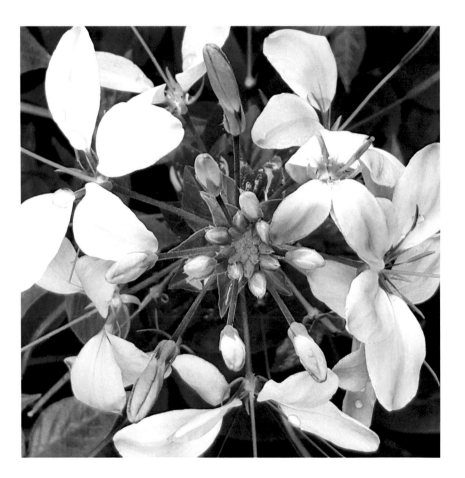

4

Practices to Cultivate Sanctuary

There is a way of breathing that's a shame and a suffocation.
And there's another way of expiring, a love breath, that lets
you open infinitely.
JALĀL AD-DĪN MUHAMMAD RŪMĪ

Practices form us. In other words, practices train us in
how to be as we move through our days.

A good practice is life-giving. Like "a love breath," it allows our soul to open wide.

Life is exquisitely better when you include at least one life-giving practice in the regular rhythm of your daily and weekly routines.

Your practice can be as simple as saying *thank you* to welcome each new day. Or it can be something more: five minutes each day to jot down who and what you're grateful for. Five minutes of being still. On purpose. Next week, bump it up to 10 minutes.

Here's what matters most: be intentional and choose a practice that delights and refreshes you. When you do, you will find it easier to commit to your practice on a regular basis.

Done regularly and with delight, your practice can make your interior life more bountiful and satisfying. As that bounty and satisfaction renews and invigorates your inner life, it will seep into your outer life.

Sanctuary speaks the language of the soul. Drawing on the soul's language, which includes gratitude, beauty, and silence, there are numerous practices from diverse contexts that cultivate sanctuary.

The practices I include here are:

Gratitude
Beauty
Silence
Music
Solitude
Being with nature
Prayer
Slowing
Reflection

I've used these practices with people of all ages in diverse contexts: aerospace, business, civic, community, education, faith-based, finance, healthcare, human services, IT, law, leadership development, military, philanthropy, political, and social justice.

As you learn about the different practices in the pages ahead, choose one practice that suits you. Try it for a while. Then add another practice.

GRATITUDE

Gratitude is the soul's way of rejoicing, a time-honored way to express our joy for the abundant blessings in our lives.

Expressing gratitude is also a way to pause and remember that each day is a precious gift.

When you express gratitude, share your joy, and celebrate your blessings, you open your heart and open the door to new possibilities and greater abundance.

Cultivate the practice of gratitude by being present to and grateful for the abundant grace, mercies, and protections in your life. Because of these bountiful blessings, you are here. Alive. Vibrant. Astonishing.

Give thanks daily. Continually. Carry this practice with you wherever you go.

Consciously cultivating thankfulness is
a journey of the soul, one that begins
when we look around us
and see the positive effects that gratitude creates.

M. J. RYAN

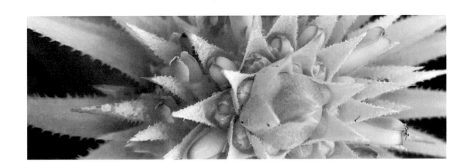

BEAUTY

Beauty is food for our soul.

As Thomas Moore reminds us, "What food is to the body, arresting, complex, and pleasing images are to the soul." And so are arresting, complex, and pleasing places, sounds, and experiences. That is why it takes our breath away to witness an exquisite persimmon sunset. To hear a beautiful, soul-stirring jazz suite by John Coltrane. To experience the awesome wonder of a solitary shooting star against a black expanse of sky.

We embrace our full humanity and divinity when we are aware of and in contact with that which is beautiful.

Remember that beauty is everywhere.

Cultivate the practice of beauty by being aware of the astonishing beauty all around you. The smile of a child. Wind whispering in the trees. First flowers that push through the warming earth after winter's long chill: yellow crocus, grape hyacinth, paper-white narcissus. The satisfying shape of a hand-thrown vase. The aroma of just-baked bread. The amazing artistry of corn-rowed hair.

Acknowledge the beauty in your life. Not just once in a while. Notice daily. As you take in beauty, your soul will become more beautiful. Our Navajo sisters and brothers encourage us to walk in beauty so that we might carry beauty with us and imbue beauty at all times.

Happily may I walk.
May it be beautiful before me.
May it be beautiful behind me.
May it be beautiful below me.
May it be beautiful above me.
May it be beautiful all around me.
In beauty it is finished.

NAVAJO PRAYER

It is the beauty within us
that makes it possible
for us to recognize the beauty around us.

JOAN CHITTISTER

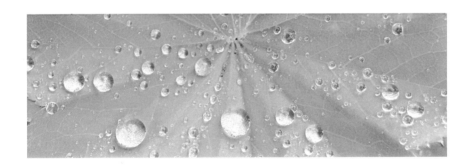

SILENCE

Silence is that gracious space where there is no activity, sound, or words.

In our noise-polluted culture, silence is not just a luxury. It is a necessity.

In silence, we hear what is essential.

In silence, we can listen for and attend to the deep desires of our own heart. As poet Rainer Maria Rilke reminds us, "Our task is to listen to the news that is always arriving out of silence."

In silence we can develop an intimacy with ourselves that is otherwise impossible.

In silence, we rest and renew ourselves emotionally, intellectually, physically, and spiritually.

Cultivate the practice of silence by turning off your cell phone, iPad, computer, TV, and video games.

Appreciate the silence.

Find a time when you will not be interrupted or distracted. And find a place—real or imaginary—to practice silence daily. Begin with 5 minutes. Next week, try 10 minutes. The following week, try 15 minutes. Then 30. Then try to practice silence for 60 minutes each day.

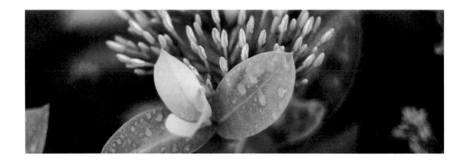

In this spacious silence, Mother Teresa reminds us…

You can hear God everywhere—in the closing
of the door, in the person who needs you,
in the birds that sing,
in the flowers, in the animals.

MOTHER TERESA

MUSIC

Throughout the ages, the art of music has held a sacred place in our lives. In our contemporary culture, music's higher purposes have been muted or forgotten. Once intended to illuminate, uplift, and assist in humanity's spiritual evolution, we now use music as a mere prop for marketing or as mundane entertainment.

But music is so much more.

Beyond being a sacred treasure, music is love and sorrow, imagination and wonder made audible.

When we create music or listen to it and honor it for the precious gifts it provides, our lives are vastly enriched.

Cultivate the practice of creating or listening to music by humming a melody you already know. Or create your own song. You can also listen to uplifting or soothing music. Try listening to music without words—instrumental music—so you aren't distracted by the message of the lyrics.

Bring instrumental music into your life daily. Or simply hum the song in your own heart.

After silence, that which comes nearest
to expressing the inexpressible
is music.

ALDOUS HUXLEY

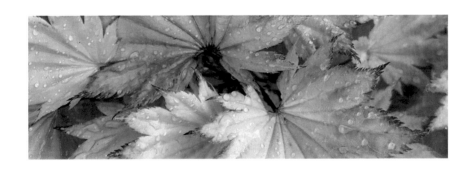

SOLITUDE

Solitude is uninterrupted time for you to be alone. Undistracted. Undisturbed.

Solitude means unplugging from your electronics—computers, tablets, and cell phones. It means getting off the grid and away from it all.

Solitude provides us with the oxygen required for deep rest, renewal, and restoration.

In solitude, your soul can open wide. You can listen deeply. You can reconnect with who you are when you are not overly identified with the roles you play at work, at school, in your family, and in your community.

Cultivate the practice of solitude by making time to be alone.

Practice being alone at least once a week. Set aside at least one hour on the same day each week. Make a date with yourself. Put it on your calendar.

Expand your weekly rhythm to include a half-day or day-long solo retreat once a month.

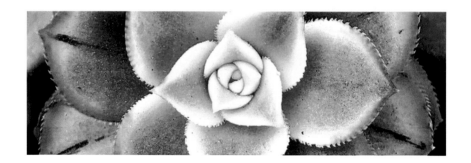

In solitude, we are silent,
so that we may hear,
focused so that we may craft
substantial things.

PAM GROUT

Solitude is the furnace of transformation.

HENRI NOUWEN

BEING WITH NATURE

If we read her closely, nature is a sacred text, a text where fiddlehead ferns, leathery oak leaves, and clouds rising from the valley floor become scripture.

In a culture that has lost sight of the sacred, being with nature offers special opportunities to:

Remember that you are part of nature.

Slow down so you can truly enjoy life at nature's pace.

Notice and enjoy the rising, noontide, and setting of the sun. The opening and closing of blossoms. Birdsong.

Notice and enjoy the rhythm of the seasons, which unfold at their own pace in their own time.

Reconnect with yourself.

Reconnect with the earth, the very ground that supports and sustains you.

Cultivate the practice of being with nature by walking barefoot in your own yard. In your neighborhood or a nearby park, pay attention to the flowers and trees. Notice the bees and butterflies. Notice the birds.

Make time daily to be with nature. Remember the birdsong, vibrant colors, and spaciousness of this time. Remember the sound of your own breathing. Tuck these treasures in your pocket so you can appreciate your oneness with nature, feeling her heartbeat as the rhythm of your daily life.

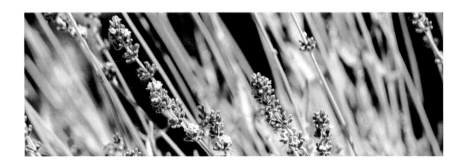

There is something infinitely healing
in the repeated refrains of nature—the assurance
that dawn comes after night,
and spring after winter.

RACHEL CARSON

PRAYER

Prayer is a posture we take towards living.

To a child, attention is love. And that kind of loving attention can be a form of prayer.

Other forms of prayer include singing, dancing, writing, gardening, and reading sacred texts. Preparing breakfast or baking bread or plowing a field with an attitude of devotion and reverence is also a form of prayer.

Rumi reminds us of rejoicing prayer when he exclaims, "There are a thousand ways to kneel and kiss the ground. There are a thousand ways to go home again."

We can go home again through prayer.

Years ago, I was in a car accident. After many, many months of healing from my injuries, I was finally able to enjoy short hikes once again on the mountain trails near my home.

On my first outing, each step and each stop became a prayer. During one extended stop, I found shaded respite in a grove of quaking aspen. Though I didn't have words for it at the time, I now realize that my mountain outing was a way to go home again, home to myself. I wrote a poem to celebrate my healing journey—"A Yellow Wood."

A Yellow Wood

Early autumn
Ascending Mount Si.
Embraced by grace
   in a yellow wood.

Generous sun
   and a blessing of gentle wind.

Stirred by shimmering,
   I lift my face
      to the slow golden dance
       of aspen leaves.

My heart restored, I am
   quickened again
     to prayer.

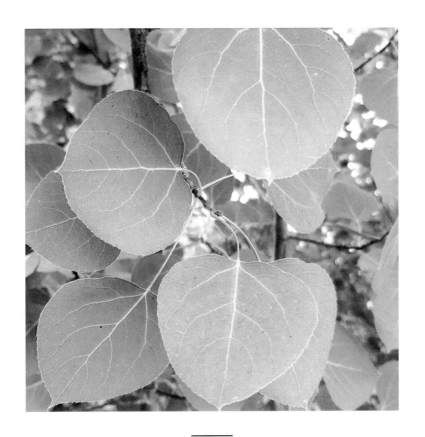

The word *prayer* comes from ancient roots. To pray for someone or something is to ask earnestly, to ask from your heart.

You can easily create your own prayer.

Pray for someone who is sick or lonely.

Pray for our service women and men.

Pray for our teachers and our youth.

Say a prayer for the food that nourishes you. This kind of prayer is also called a blessing or grace.

Cultivate the practice of prayer by entering into a relationship with what is most sacred to you: caring for your family, preparing a meal, planting a garden of herbs, journaling about your day.

Make prayer part of your daily routine. Consider each conversation a form of prayer.

> *Prayer is not doing, but being.*
> *It is not the words but the beyond-words experience*
> *of coming into the presence of something*
> *much greater than oneself.*
> KATHLEEN NORRIS

SLOWING

Slowing is a deliberate act of refusal.

When you slow down, you refuse busyness and hurry. You refuse reactivity. You refuse your need to be in control.

Instead, you can make positive, life-affirming agreements. Choose to be still. Choose to be present to yourself and others. Choose to listen. Choose to be centered instead of scattered and unfocused.

The purpose of slowing is to restore balance in your life, and to center you in being fully present.

Cultivate the practice of slowing by deliberately choosing stillness. For 5 minutes each day.

In this stillness, devote yourself to breathing. Begin by slowly taking in a deep breath. Then slowly exhale. Do it again. Repeat 10 times.

After a week, add this to your slowing practice: as you take a deep breath, breathe in slowness and breathe out busyness. Practice for 5 minutes each day for a month. Practice again next month. This time, breathe in peace, breathe out hurry. Next month, breathe in harmony, breathe out chaos.

Change your slowing practice each month. In a year, you will have transformed your life.

Carry your slowing practice with you wherever you go.

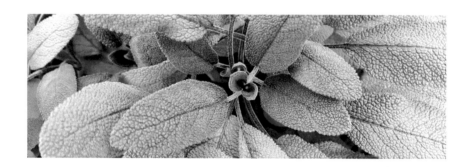

Slowing is a way we counter our culture's mandate to tend to the bottom line, to move it or lose it, to constantly be on the go.

ADELE CALHOUN

REFLECTION

Reflection gives us a reason to stop, shine the light on and savor our experiences, and look at them with fresh eyes. It provides us the opportunity to chew on, metabolize, and make meaning of our experiences.

On the way to making meaning, reflection opens us to an expanse of wilderness, allowing us to experience ripples and waves of wonder and awe.

Cultivate the practice of reflection by focusing on a favorite quote or proverb or song or poem. Read or review it to yourself. Silently at first, then aloud. Choose a word or phrase that stands out to you. Stop. Let that word or phrase settle in your heart. Reflect on it. Meditate on it. What other words or phrases or music or images or experiences does it bring forth?

Whatever emerges, jot it down on a slip of paper. For one week, notice where it appears in your life.

Now, notice for a month. Looking back on your life, where has this word or phrase or image appeared before? Is there any connection to who you are now and who you are becoming?

Reflection is a powerful,
dynamic process that ushers in
learning and points the way
to new possibilities.

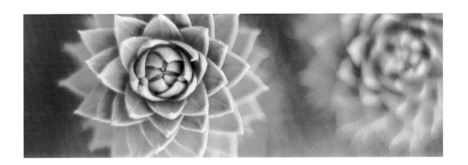

Notes

Notes

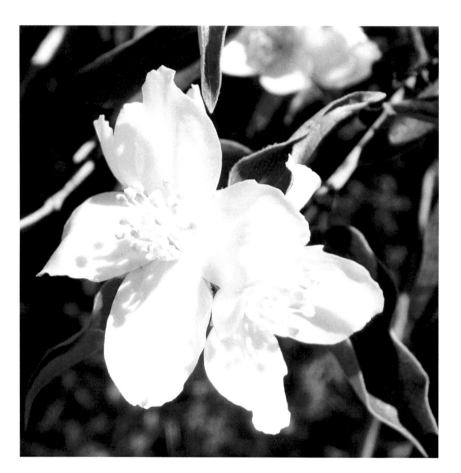

Grace Notes

Ultimately, we seek, make way for, and cultivate practices so that sanctuary might become more deeply ingrained in our daily routine. So that sanctuary might become a way to live. A way to live that restores the rhythm of rest and renewal in our lives, creating the conditions for us to enter into *Kairos*—that extraordinary experience of the eternal—anytime, anywhere.

blessing the light
(thinking of Lucille Clifton)

may the stars
that shimmer even now
beneath the surface of our knowing
light your way
beyond the valley of fear
may you open your arms
then pull them back
assured that another's will shelter you
from any storm   may you
lift your face to the sun
sun that favors you always
and may you in your brilliance shine
          a beacon for others from here to there

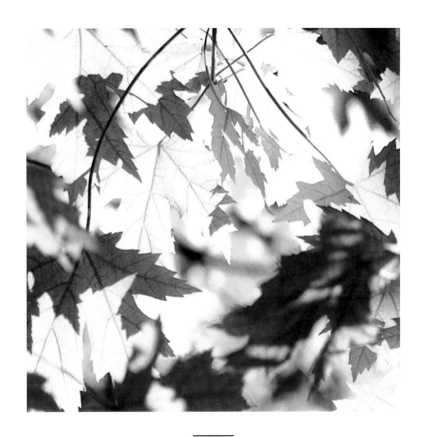

Notes

Notes

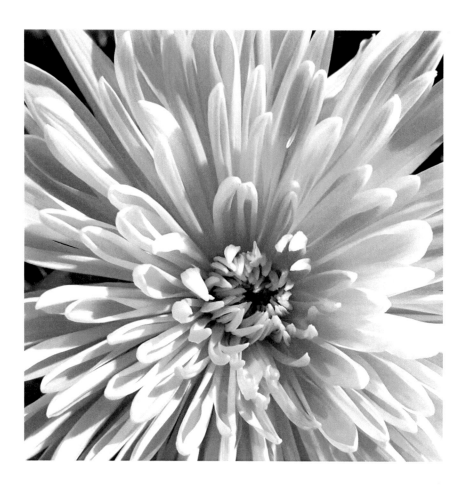

About the Author

Gloria J. Burgess is a writer, speaker, poet, and activist. Her focus is social transformation through spirit-filled leadership, arts, and education. As CEO of Jazz International and Executive Director of The Lift Every Voice Foundation, she leads both organizations to inspire, develop, and equip leaders throughout the world.

Gloria holds a PhD from the University of Southern California and is a Distinguished Scholar in Performance Studies and

Theatre. She is also a Cave Canem Poetry Fellow, a prestigious collective of poets and writers of the African diaspora.

Gloria has written eight books, including *Flawless Leadership, Dare to Wear Your Soul on the Outside*, *Legacy Living*, and *Pass It On!*, her beautifully illustrated book about her father's life-changing friendship with Nobel Laureate William Faulkner.

A former executive in IT, human services, and philanthropy, Gloria serves as strategic catalyst and speaker, impacting hundreds of thousands of people in diverse contexts: Microsoft, Starbucks, AT&T, Boeing, Bill & Melinda Gates Foundation, Girl Scouts of America, Casey Family Programs, International Coach Federation, Kenya's Parliament, South African Embassy, and Paraguay's Office of the President. She is also a professor in executive leadership at Seattle University, University of Washington, and University of Southern California.

Gloria leads private and public workshops on *Sanctuary*. Book your workshop today: Events@gloriaburgess.com.

Learn more about Gloria's work at www.gloriaburgess.com or contact gloria@gloriaburgess.com.

Gloria lives in the Pacific Northwest overlooking the beautiful waters of the Salish Sea.

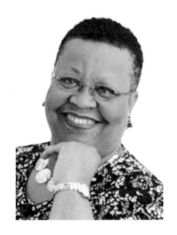